The Best Crude Food Recipes

By

Aliona Ann

Table of contents

Salsa And Evening Bites

Salsa
Cucumber With Goat Cheddar
Avocado Coleslaw
Tapenade
Petso
Zucchini Hummus
Pecan Pate

Super

Pizza
Spaghetti Al Pesto Or Marinara
Portobello Mushroom Steak
Mexican Meat Portion Recipe For Tortillas
Tortillas
Crude French Fries Recipe
Ketchup
Crude Broccoli Salad
Salad Potato
Lasagna

Treats, Cake And Pastry

Energy Bars
Frozen yogurt
Vanilla cream

Crude Food Essentials

The Most Effective Method To Eat Yourself Sound

It is easy to Eat food. Be that as it may, eating straightforward is quite possibly the most troublesome thing today. There isn't enough regular spring water accessible to all. Furthermore, we can't process crude wild green grasses and plants any longer. Also, there is allurement of modest low quality food all over the place.

Low quality food isn't normal. Regular alone will persevere. Regular eating has persevered for millennia. While never burning through billions of dollars on advertising. Eating straightforwardly and regularly is just the presence of mind. A mistake doesn't become truth due to continued promoting. Nor does truth become a mistake since no one sees it.

What you eat consistently communicates your needs. Is your need to be solid, vigorous and blissful? Make the world a superior spot? Or on the other hand do you like to not think or plan, destroy Television at home, remain in your usual range of familiarity, and be acknowledged and preferred by others. This is what you need to ask yourself. What is your actual need? Choose and live by it.

Your need is your objective. To remind yourself everyday and persuade yourself to seek after it, compose your own objective down a paper and stick it on your refrigerator, make it your PC secret key, set a caution in your schedule to remind you routinely, post a moving statement or picture in your restroom or mirror, read books about the subject, pay attention to tapes, watch DVDs and go to gatherings where the subject of your objective is talked about. Separate your objective in little and simple ways to do ordinary errands. Then go.

To remain propelled I have a spot in my kitchen with crude cheap food to remind me and make it simple for me to eat along these lines: green powder, superfood blends, crude chocolate bar, natural product, trail blends, energy bars, decontaminated water. I have pictures of motivating sound individuals on my PC and in my restroom. My PC secret phrase incorporated the word sound. I read books on crude food, go to crude food occasions, welcome individuals over to attempt crude food (like juice or chocolate gatherings and potlucks), compose on my site http://www.thebestofrawfood.com , do research, converse with individuals in the crude food stores and so forth.

My need is being solid and cheerful so you can help your family, companions and other intrigued individuals to become sound and blissful as well. Subsequent to exploring, noticing and encountering, I accept that eating a characteristic eating regimen is basic to arriving. To me a normal solid eating regimen is one that comprises generally crude, plant based and supplement thick food.

In this book you will find recipes that are made with these fixings. Are not difficult to get ready first off of a crude food diet and are extraordinarily delightful. This way it is not difficult to remain propelled and continue to go.

What To Eat

I like to eat food uncooked on the grounds that when it's crude, it is loaded with chemicals, effectively absorbable minerals and life force. Food is viewed as crude in the event that it is rarely warmed over 42 C/118 F degrees. Furthermore, I like it as new (and wild) as could really be expected. What's more, obviously liberated from additives, pesticides, light what's more, hereditary control. Center around the accompanying nutrition classes:

1. Green verdant vegetables

2. Ocean Vegetables (Nori, Kelp, Dulse, Irish Mosh, and so on.)

3. (Wild) Spices and Flavors (for example Basil, Stevia, Garlic, Cilantro, Ginger, Stew Pepper, Mint).

4. Restorative Mushrooms (for example Shiitake, Maitake, Reishi, Chaga).

5. Super food sources (= food that supplement thick): for example crude chocolate, goji berries, youthful coconut water, green powders.

6. Wheatgrass and Fledglings.

7. Seeds (flax, hemp, chia, sesame, pumpkin, sunflower).

8. Food matured with support of biotics: for example (uncooked) sauerkraut, pickles, refreshments, miso.

9. Spotless and amazing drinking water.
In this book you will track down models on the most proficient method to utilize these fixings to make scrumptious, satisfying and simple to plan feasts. Eating them will support your energy like you have never experienced previously.

Join these food sources with a casual way of life, blissful considerations and being straightforwardly grounded to the earth. Uncover your skin and eyes to some immediate daylight consistently and marvels may occur.

How To Plan

You can essentially eat a similar diet on a crude food diet as you would on a cooked eating routine. What is the most striking contrast, other than de-fixing, is the planning of your food. The following arrangement techniques are to:

1. Guarantee that your food stays under 42 C/118 F degrees
2. Get a favored consistency
3. Make your food effectively absorbable or potentially
4. Save your food

Arrangement Techniques

Here are the most involved arrangement techniques for making crude food dishes.
1. Squeezing
2. Mixing
3. Drying out
4. Cutting

Squeezing

Squeezing is a method for getting the fluid (juice) out of a vegetable or natural product. The fiber is taken out, the juice is left. This is a method for getting concentrated nutrients and minerals that are very simple for your body to ingest. The supplements might enter your circulation system in 20 minutes or less.
There are three sort of juicers:
1. Citrus juicers (squeezed orange);
2. Axis juicers (carrots);
3. "Slow" juicers (greens).

Citrus juicers are the ones you use for lemons and oranges. You can get some hand juicers for around 5 USD. I have a modest glass one I use for rapidly squeezing lemon juice.

Axis juicers are speedy and simple to utilize. They function admirably for more earnestly products of the soil like apples, carrots, cucumber, celery, ginger, beets. You can likewise involve them for entire lemons and oranges (stripped!). You might attempt to place in certain greens,however they don't get a lot of juice out of them. They range in cost from 50 - 500 USD. I like the Solis or Breville brand.

Slow Juicers are best utilized for green verdant vegetables and grasses. In any case, they likewise work for apples, carrots and cucumbers. They are the most costly, by and large are more work to juice (may need to be pre-cut) and to clean. In any case, they are stopped and remove the most squeeze.

Additionally, they for the most part give you the best quality juice and supplements in view of added magnets as well as a gentler method for treating the product.

Mixing

Mixing is a method for cutting produce so little that it turns into a smooth soup, or "smoothie". Excellent rapid blenders, for example, Blendtec and Vitamix cut the food so minuscule that the cell wall is broken. This makes it simple for you to assimilate extreme vegetables. Mixing utilizes the entire food, subsequently the fiber remains.

You can mix organic products, vegetables, greens, super food sources, water, nuts, seeds, and so on. You can make cold or warm smoothies, sweet or generous.

Blenders are extremely simple being used and fast to clean. An extremely well known method for getting ready crude food. My most memorable crude food year I utilized a hand blender (700 watt).

Moderately economical and it functioned admirably I actually utilize one when I travel. Clearly, it doesn't make the food as smooth (particularly greens like spinach) and it won't break the cell mass of greens so it isn't as simple to retain the smoothies.
Vitamix and Blendec are the best blenders. They are truly a venture yet definitely justified since you will utilize them frequently.

Getting dried out

Getting dried out is a method for drying your food and taking the water out. Once dried out, you can store your food in an impermeable holder or plastic sack. It is likewise a method for making the food crunchy and frequently utilized as an option in contrast to ordinary baking.

However, since the food ought to stay "crude" it can't be dried out in an ordinary broiler. Best ways of getting dried out are to allow the food to sun dry or utilize a unique dehydrator (for example Excalibur).

Alternate ways are to utilize your radiator or your regular stove on the most reduced temperature.

Assuming that you might want to make luxurious cuisine, I would absolutely get one. In any case, this machine wouldn't be on the first spot on my list. It's huge, costly and getting dried out at low temperatures takes for the most part 6 - 24 hours for your food to be prepared.

Cutting

You can cut your food with sharp knives, a shaper, mandoline or food processor.
Sharp knives are significant while planning crude food and obviously a cutting board.

A hand shaper is simple when you really want to cut numerous onions or nuts. It's a problem to clean them.

A food processor is great to make a pesto. In this way something not totally smooth (which it will get assuming you placed it in your blender) or for utilizing more modest amounts. I use my hand blender for this and heartbeat, or utilize the food processor part of my hand blender. I would just involve a food processor for bigger amounts. (I by and large get ready crude nourishment for just 1 or 2 individuals).

A mandoline is for no particular reason. You can make pleasant shapes, for example, potato shapes, ribs, or very slender cuts. Moderately economical and ideal to have, yet all the same not an unquestionable requirement.

What Food To Pick

To plan tasty and good feasts, pick the best food. This will gigantically influence the progress of your dish. Particularly, search for natural, new and nearby if you can.

Since you are involving new items the recommended fixings in the fixings rundown of the recipes might need to be changed by the size or wellspring of the food.

A tip: thus, begin with just a portion of how much the recorded elements of flavors that are zesty or solid, for example, cayenne pepper or ginger. Taste and afterward add more assuming you like.

This way you keep away from that you will "ruin" your dish with an excess of ginger or garlic.

Food Handling

While planning crude food it's essential to be sterile and store your edibles securely.

1. Be cautious with cutting sheets, knives and plates and clean up previously getting ready and eating your dinners.

2. Purchase just food sources from sources you trust.

3. Refrigerate your food.

4. Try not to avoid edibles with regard to the cooler for over two hours (particularly the pate's, nut milks and creature food varieties).

5. You can utilize food grade hydrogen peroxide to sanitize your food (1 drop is more successful than cooking).

6. Try not to eat in cafés, where you don't have any idea and where food isn't ready before your eyes, cleanliness is drilled stringently or where not many individuals come to eat..

The Recipes

The recipes in this book are arranged by when to eat them. In this manner. breakfast, lunch, supper, bites and beverages. (However, clearly, you can have a lunch recipe for supper or the other way around).

Begin your morning with a crude food breakfast and work up until every one of your feasts are crude.

Your body will be appreciative to such an extent that it will get the fuel to recuperate and clean itself. Creatures will be much obliged to you since you let them carry on with a decent life and the planet will see the value in you eating a crude natural (for the most part) plant based diet that will really recover the earth.

What's more, Gandhi would have said thanks to you for "Being the change you need to find on the planet". Much obliged to you for pursuing this book. I wish you a phenomenal expansion in wellbeing, excellence and bliss.

Crude Food Breakfast

Oat Dinner

Serves 2

Fixings
2 apples
1 banana
1 tablespoon brilliant flax seed
2 teaspoons cinnamon decontaminated water

Bearings

1. Put the flax seeds in the decontaminated water and let sit for the time being.

2. Strip the apples and cut them into little pieces (for the blender).

3. Strip the banana and break it into parts. Flush the flax seeds.

4. Put all fixings in a blender. This can be a hand blender or high velocity blender like Vitamix.

5. Add 1⁄4 cup water, to allow the combination to mix well.

6. Mix all fixings until smooth. You might need to add some more water assuming it's as well thick.

Tips
•You make this recipe far and away superior by supplanting the water with almond cream or new juice. You may likewise add a tablespoon of hemp seeds. My little girl likes to add (sprouted) nuts and raisins.

•You can sct up this recipe the prior night (however put the banana in there in the morning). Particularly with nuts and dried natural products in it, it will just taste better!

Vanilla Yogurt

Serves 1

Fixings
1/2 cup coconut water
1 cup coconut meat
1/2 teaspoon vanilla concentrate

Bearings

1. Open the coconut with a knife.

2. Pour the coconut water in the container of a high velocity blender and some or the
the entirety of the milk.

3. Mix well. You ought to get the consistency of yogurt.

Tips
•You can drink it for all intents and purposes or you can add a product of your decision. Consider peach, strawberries, mango or pear. So great!
•A phenomenal replacer of yogurt produced using dairy. It's scrumptious as a yogurt dessert, for breakfast with granola or you can place it in your ice producer machine and you get scrumptious frozen yogurt.

Apple Avocado Mousse

Serves 2

Fixings

1 avocado
2 apples
1/4 cup decontaminated water

Bearings

1.Ring the apples and take out the center.
2.Remove the avocado meat from the avocado.
3.Put the two fixings in a bowl. Blend well in with a hand blender.

Energy Bomb Smoothie

This is my number one crude breakfast recipe. I drink this smoothie each day, or a variety of it is great and very filling! A dietary bomb! Loaded with minerals, chemicals, co-factors furthermore, excellent protein.

I can utilize a smidgen of crude chocolate and I could live on only these smoothies. I drink just

2 every day and afterward a plate of mixed greens around evening time. The crude chocolate is an extraordinary replacer for espresso.

At the point when you utilize warm water or tea (not warmed over 170 F) you have a decent warm beverage.

Fixings

1 teaspoon of crude carob powder (or crude chocolate)
1 tablespoon goji berries
1/2 teaspoon maca powder
1 teaspoon honey bee dust
1 tablespoon hemp seed
1 teaspoon crude honey (or yacon root or not many drops stevia)
1 teaspoon green powder (spirulina, chlorella, wheat grass)
not many leafs of greens (like spinach or dandelion)
barely any scoops of coconut meat (discretionary)
2 cups extraordinary warm spice tea or unadulterated water or coconut water

Bearings

1.Blend all in a blender and appreciate it!

Mango Smoothie

This mango smoothie makes an eminent breakfast and gives sufficient energy to last an entire morning. It's a crude and veggie lover. No additional sugars dairy free.

Fixings

1 mango
2 bananas
1-2 oranges
run of lemon juice
1 tablespoon hemp seed
1/4 teaspoon green powder
ice 3D shapes (discretionary)

Bearings

1. Strip and pit the mango, cut into pieces.

2. Strip and cut the banana and orange.

3. Put all fixings in the blender (orange first). Mix all fixings well.

Tips

•You might need to add a little water in the event that it's excessively thick. The hemp seeds give great fats, super protein and strands. This smoothie is additionally delectable with some coconut meat or water (rather than the hemp and orange).

•I frequently keep frozen mango or potentially banana in the ice chest. This way I generally have the fixings with me for making this recipe.

Hemp and Berry Smoothie

Serves 2

Fixings

1 Banana
2 Tablespoons hulled hemp seed
1 Pack of frozen berries
1 Cup unadulterated water

Headings

1. Put all fixings in a fast blender.

2. Add sufficient water with the goal that all fixings are covered. Mix well. You probably will need to add somewhat more water assuming that it's excessively thick. You might mix longer assuming you think that it is excessively cold.

Tips
•The hemp seeds give great fats and super protein.

•Hemp seeds are the main seeds that have no compound inhibitor and consequently don't have to absorb water prior to eating.

•On the off chance that the berries are sharp, you might add a couple of drops of (fluid) stevia to the smoothie to get a better taste.

Lunch

Guacamole

Serves 3

Fixings

3 avocados, pitted
1 onion, diced
2 tomatoes, diced
2 branches new cilantro, finely slashed 1 lime or lemon
2 cloves garlic cayenne pepper to taste ocean salt to taste
1/2 cup refined water

Bearings

1. Scoop the meat from the avocado skin.

2. Cut the avocados into pieces, place in an enormous bowl, and pound with a spoon.

3. Delicately mix in the onions, tomatoes and cilantro.

4. Crush in the lime squeeze and mix in salt to taste.

Tips

•Totally wonderful with (independent) flax seed saltines, grew bread (for example Ezenkiel) or on the other hand the rosemary wafers from Unadulterated Food and Wine/1 fortunate duck.

•Extraordinary as a plunge for crudités (carrots, celery, broccoli, ringer peppers)

Flax Seed Saltines

Serves 4

Fixings

1 cup ground flax sccd
1/4 cup sesame seeds
1/4 cup buckwheat
1 or 2 handful dried natural product (raisins, goji berries, cut of figs)
1/2 tablespoon ocean salt
1 cup water

Bearings

1. Blend all dry fixings in a bowl.

2. Add the water. Blend once more.

3. Let represent no less than 2 hours with the goal that the sugar from the natural product can be imbued and doused by the seeds. You might need to mix periodically to check whether there is sufficient water. It's not in any way important to drench when you utilize ground flax seeds (as gone against entire flax seeds) however I find the saltines taste much better on the off chance that you do.

4. Spread the player uniformly on a plate. I use a broiler plate with Teflon or silicone sheets,a dehydrator plate with Teflon sheets, you could in fact utilize an enormous clay plate (yet put some coconut oil on the base so it will fall off without any problem). You can spread the hitter with the rear of a spoon, a spatula or with your hands.

5. Presently, how about we dry out. You can do this in a dehydrator, ordinary stove at most

reduced setting and ideally one that can be placed on dry air, direct daylight, on top of a radiator. The key is that the temperature of the food ought not be raised over 40 degrees Celsius or 115 Fahrenheit. A food thermometer (utilized for hamburgers!) may help you decide this.

6. Hold on until the top is dried well. In the sun and customary broiler is around 2 hours. In the dehydrator around 4 hours, contingent upon how much water was added to the player.

7. Then flip and let it dry out for one more hour.

Tips
•You can eat the saltines warm or cold. On the off chance that it dried well, you can store the saltines in a compartment that will keep any wet out. (it's dry when there is no consolidate in the shut compartment)

•These saltines are perfect for lunch with avocado, pesto and tomato. You can add some other spread .

•Likewise extraordinary as a bite, or as chips. Simply modify this essential recipe.

•What's perfect about these flax seed recipes with saltines is that the varieties are boundless. Explore different avenues regarding adding different seeds, for example, hemp seed, or nuts (pecan, brazil, almond).

•Or then again take a stab at adding other dried natural products, like dates or apricots, even olives or dried tomatoes (cut them in little pieces and allow them to drench with the seeds). You might need to eliminate the salt assuming that you use olives or dried tomatoes since they are pungent by
themselves.

•In the event that you make the saltines somewhat thicker and eat them warm, they really taste to some degree like bread. (be that as it may, much better)

Lettuce Wraps

Serves 4

Fixings

1/2 cup hemp seed
1/2 cup lemon juice
1/4 cup honey or a couple of drops of stevia (2-
3)
1 1/2 tablespoon cleaved ginger
1/2 tablespoon red stew
1 tablespoon soy sauce
1 cup crude almond spread
1/2 head savoy cabbage, destroyed
6 exceptionally huge wild spinach leafs
1 carrot
1 ready mango
1 small bunch cilantro leafs
1 small bunch torn basil leafs
Himalaya ocean salt

Bearings
1. Cut the carrot into matchstick-size pieces.

2. Cut the Mango longwise into strips, around
1/4 inch (1 cm) thick.

3. In a Vita-Blend or rapid blender, purée the
honey (or stevia), lemon juice, ginger, red bean
stew, and soy sauce.

4. Add the almond margarine and mix at low speed to join. You ought to get a fairly thick consistency. (You might add water assuming it should be more slender).

5. In a bowl, blend the almond spread dressing with the cabbage. The best and most straightforward way is to do this with your hands or a huge wooden spoon.

6. Presently you want to fold the cabbage with dressing into a "lettuce" wrap. This is somewhat interesting. Put the spinach leaf on a cutting block with the underside confronting.

7. Then, at that point, you put a portion of the cabbage blend on the leaf.

8. Add some hemp seeds, a couple of sticks of carrot, a couple of bits of mango, and a couple of leaves of cilantro and basil.

9. Attempt to move up and the spinach leaf, you could have to put a mixed drink stick in it to hold. Do this for the wide range of various spinach leaves until the fixings are no more.

Tips

This is my outright most loved lunch dish. It's an adjusted and improved form of Unadulterated Food and Wine's "Thai Lettuce Wraps". Assuming you at any point go to NY, I energetically suggest you attempt them in this café. In the event that you carry this dish to a lunch or potluck, you'll be wowed!

As an option in contrast to assembling the wraps yourself, it's entirely enjoyable to let your visitors set up the actual wrap. This will save you time and it adds to a social extraordinary air of your supper

On the off chance that you live in the US, you can likewise utilize collard greens rather than the spinach leaves, yet I haven't tracked down them in the Netherlands yet.

Tomato And Olive Serving Of Mixed Greens

Serves 4

Fixings
4 sections cherry tomatoes 1 section olives
crude additional virgin olive oil
lemon juice to taste
ocean salt and pepper to taste
modest bunch basil
arugula or different greens (discretionary)

Headings

1. Break the tomatoes with the goal that the juice emerges (best in a cup so squeeze won't spill)

2. Consolidate the tomatoes and olives in a bowl.

3. Add the olive oil, lemon squeeze and pepper.

4. Throw.

5. Not long before supper, add the basil and arugula.

Thai Coleslaw

Serves 4

Fixings

1/2 cup crude cashews
1/2 cup lemon juice
2 tablespoons hacked ginger
1/2 tablespoon red stew
1 1/2 tablespoon tamari
1 cup crude almond or peanut butter
1/2 head white cabbage, destroyed
1/4 cup red cabbage, destroyed
1/4 cup carrots, destroyed
1 ready mango, cut in little dices
1 small bunch cilantro leafs
1 small bunch torn basil leafs
2 tablespoons of honey (or supplant with not many drops stevia)
Himalaya ocean salt

Headings

1.Cut the mango into little shapes.

2.Shred the cabbage and carrots.

3.In a rapid blender, purée the honey, lemon juice, ginger, red bean stew and tamari.

4.Add the crude almond margarine and mix at low speed to consolidate. To get a thick, cakehitter like consistency.
5.Add water to thin if essential.

6.In a bowl blend the cabbage and the crude almond spread combination all around well.

7.Add the crude cashews and mango pieces.

8.Top with leaves of cilantro and basil and a couple of bits of mango as well as carrots for variety.

Avocado Carrot Soup

Serves 2

Fixings
1 Avocado
1 Medium carrot
1/4 Cup almond (hemp or sesame) Milk

1 Tablespoon ginger (finely cleaved)
1/2 Lemon
2-4 Drops liquid stevia or 1 tablespoon of crude honey (discretionary)
Squeeze cayenne pepper
Unadulterated Water

Headings

1.Put all fixings in a rapid blender and blend
 well.

2.Add some filtered water or carrot juice would be a good idea for you like a thicker consistency.

Tip
•Tasty as plunge or soup

Kelp Salad

Fixings

Kelp of your decision (crude, unroasted) stevia
Crude sesame oil
Sesame seeds

Tamari lemon juice

Bearings

1. For the dressing: consolidate stevia, oil, soy and lemon juice.

2. Blend in with the ocean growth.

3. Sprinkle sesame seeds on top.

Gazpacho

Serves 4

Fixings
4 tomatoes, diced
1 medium white onion, diced
2 garlic cloves, stripped and minced
3 cups refined water
crude apple juice vinegar to taste
lemon juice to taste
1 cucumber, stripped and slashed
4 tablespoons newly slashed cilantro (discretionary)
1 scallion (green part), finely slashed, for embellish

1 red chime pepper, cultivated, cored, and diced
(discretionary)
1 tablespoon crude virgin olive oil
1/4 cup mango, diced in little 3D shapes

Headings

1. Place the tomatoes, onion, garlic, water,
vinegar, lemon juice, cucumber and cilantro in a
blender and purée.

2. Strain (vegetable press is least demanding) to
eliminate any vegetable pieces and pits that are
not completely melted. (in the event that you
have a juicer, you can likewise place all fixings
in the juicer,utilizing a coarse screen).

3. Chill for the time being, assuming time
licenses.

4. Prior to serving, sprinkle the slashed
scallions, olive oil, some finely cut cilantro and

5. Mango over the gazpacho.

Tip

•Instead of red ringer pepper, mango and cilantro, you could likewise utilize pesto (as a beating).

Salsa And Evening Bites

Incredible with flax seed saltines, Ezekiel bread or the rosemary wafers of Unadulterated Food and Wine. Likewise a brilliant plunge for carrots, celery, broccoli and ringer peppers.

Salsa

Makes around 1 1/2 cups

Fixings

1/2 green chime pepper, cultivated, cored and diced 2 tomatoes
1/2 onion, diced
1 garlic clove, hacked
2 twigs new cilantro, slashed little
juice of 1/4 lemon
1/4 cup cold-squeezed olive oil
ocean salt, to taste
slashed jalapeño pepper, to taste

Bearings

1. Consolidate the pepper, tomato, onion, garlic, cilantro, lemon squeeze and oil in a medium bowl, and throw to mix completely.

2. Season with salt and jalapeño to taste.

Cucumber With Goat Cheddar

Fixings

1 English cucumber
New delicate Goat Cheddar

Bearings

1. Cut the cucumber and spread with goat cheddar, hummus or any of the other spreads. (Additionally incredible with smoked salmon)

Avocado ColeSlaw

Serves 4

Fixings

1 cup destroyed red cabbage

1 cup destroyed green cabbage

1/2 carrot, destroyed

1 lemon (squeezed)

1 garlic cloves, minced

1 tablespoon entire grain mustard

1 avocado, pitted.

1/2 cup refined water

Headings

1. Combine the cabbage and carrot as one in an enormous bow.

2. Blend the avocado, mustard, garlic and lemon juice in a blender until smooth.

3. Pour the dressing over the serving of mixed greens and throw.

Tips

•You can set up the cabbage and carrot in enormous amounts and save in the cooler for a couple of days. Then you'll continuously have some prepared for a fast plate of mixed greens. To plan, just to add a dressing.

Tapenade

Serves 6-8

Fixings

1 clove garlic
1 cup dark olives (Qualities First Regulation
Italian)
ocean salt and pepper to taste
olive oil
juice of 1 lemon to taste

Bearings

1.Remove the pits from the olives. (if vital)

2. Place garlic, olives, olive oil and a few juices
in a blender and mix. (I lean toward not as well
fine)

3. Add salt and pepper and lemon juice to taste
and add a more olive oil to make it overall quite
smooth

Pesto

Makes around 3/4 cup

Fixings

2 tablespoons pine nuts (drenched 20 min)
6 tablespoons additional virgin olive oil
3 cloves garlic, cleaved
6 tablespoons slashed new basil
1 tablespoon slashed parsley
squeeze ocean salt

Headings

1. In a blender, join all the fixings.

2. Mix until smooth.

3. In the event that the sauce is excessively thick, add a spoonful of warm watcr.

Zucchini Hummus

Serves 2

Fixings

1 zucchini, stripped and slashed (around 1 1/2 cups)
2 tablespoons crude tahini
1/2 lemon squeezed
1 teaspoon crushed garlic (2 gloves)
1/4 teaspoon ground cumin
cayenne pepper to taste
ocean salt to taste

Headings

1.Remove the pits from the olives (if important).

2. Place garlic, olives, olive oil and a few juices in a blender and mix (I favor not as well fine).

3. Add salt and pepper and lemon juice to taste.

Pecan Pate

Makes around 1 cup

Fixings
1 cup doused crude pecans
1 tablespoon new lemon juice
1 teaspoon extra-virgin olive oil

1 teaspoon crude soy sauce
1/4 teaspoon garlic powder
run ocean salt
1 tablespoon minced new parsley
1 tablespoon minced onion

Bearings

1. Place the pecans, lemon juice, olive oil, soy sauce, garlic powder, and salt in a food processor fitted with an S cutting edge and cycle into a glue. Stop at times to scratch down the sides of the bowl with an elastic spatula.

2. Move to a little blending bowl.

3. Mix in the parsley and onion and blend well.

Supper

Pizza

Serves 4-6

Fixings
For the hull:
4 cups pecans, drenched 1 hour or more
4 cups zucchini, ground
1/2 cup brilliant flaxseed, ground
Salt and pepper, oregano, cayenne pepper to taste

Bearings

1. Beat the pecans in a food processor or hack into little pieces (like couscous), however not totally smooth and move the nuts to a huge bowl.
2. Add the zucchini, flaxseed, salt and around 1/4 cup of water, mixing to join.

3. Add more water until a tacky batter structures. You might require pretty much water.

4. Split the margarine between four 14 - inch Teflex-lined dehydrator plates.

5. Utilizing an offset spatula, spread the mixture to the edges of the plate. The mixture can be a piece sticky and tacky, so it assists with plunging the spatula in water as you spread the mixture (the abundance of water will all vanish in the dehydrator).

6. Dry out the flatbread at 115 F for 6-8 hours, or short-term. At the point when the tops are dry, flip them over and strip away the Teflex liners. Dry out on evaluates for another 2-4 hours.

7. When the two sides are dry, slide the flatbread onto a huge cutting board.

8. With an enormous gourmet expert's blade, cut into pizza rounds of your favored size and shape.

9. Put them back on the dehydrator plate and get dried out one more hour or more, as essential for firm hulls.

Fixings

For the premise:
4 cups hemp seeds
1/2 cup lemon juice
2 little cloves garlic
1/4 cup sesame tahini
1 teaspoon ocean salt
1 cup sifted water

Headings

1.In a food processor, add the nuts, lemon juice, garlic, tahini, and salt.
2.Process, adding water 1/4 cup at a time until you get the smoothie, soft consistency of hummus.
3.You might have to add more water, or you might need to add olive oil for a more extravagant hummus - simply ensure it has sufficient firmness so it will hold the fixings on the pizza without running off the sides of the outside.

Fixings

For the garnish
1 16 ounces cherry tomatoes, divided
1/4 of enormous bulb of fennel, shaved extremely meager on a mandolin
1/2 English cucumber, stripped, cultivated, and finely diced
1/2 cup Green Olive Tapenade
1/2 cup green olives, pitted and divided

Headings
1. Spread each outside layer with hummus and top with tomatoes, cucumber, olive tapenade also, olives.

Tips
•Rather than the hummus and fixing portrayed above, you can likewise spread the covering with crude goat cheddar, pesto, tomato, olives, tapenade or potentially sun dried tomato tapenade

Spaghetti Al Pesto Or Marinara

Serves 4-6

Fixings
3 pounds of yellow summer squash/zucchini

Pesto or marinara sauce:
Beating
1/4 cup olives, slashed
1/4 cup tomatoes, slashed
1/4 cup red ringer peppers, hacked 1/4 cup red onions, slashed

Headings

1. Daintily cut the yellow squash/zucchini with a sharp blade or mandolin to make strands of "pasta". Put away.

2. For the pesto/marinara sauce put all fixings in a blender and mix until smooth.

3. Throw the sauce with the cut or spiraled squash pasta and serve.

Portobello Mushroom Steak

Serves 2

Fixings
2 Portobello mushroom
2 tbsp olive oil
ocean salt and pepper to taste

Bearings

1. Clear off the mushrooms with a paper fabric or mushroom brush (don't utilize water).

2. Throw all fixings together in a bowl. Blend well.

3. Let marinate for 5-10 minutes.

4. Put in a dehydrator, (sweltering air) broiler (max 50C/120F degrees), in the sun or on your (warmed) radiator for around 1-2 hours or until delicate.

5. Eat right away (incredible when actually warm) It's simply simple! Appreciate.

Tips
•In the event that you serve it warm, it resembles having a cooked dish!

•You might act for what it's worth or you could add a few marinated onions, hacked tomato blocks, parsley for improvement.

•Next time, have a go at adding crude tamari (gluten free soy sauce), garlic, lemon as well as cayenne pepper to the marinade.

Mexican Meat Portion Recipe For Tortillas

Fixings

1 cup pecans - drenched for 2 hours
1 cup sun dried tomatoes - drenched for 60 minutes
Mexican spice combination (ground cumin, cayenne pepper)
1 inch bean stew pepper (eliminate the seeds on the off chance that you could do without it excessively hot)
1 ready tomato
olive oil
1 teaspoon tamari
2 drops stevia (or 1 tbsp honey, maple syrup)
small bunch new cilantro leafs

Bearings
1 .Put all fixings with the exception of tomato, onions and cilantro in a food processor and blend well.

2. Cut onions, tomato and cilantro in little pieces.

3. Put all fixings in a bowl. Blend in with a fork until very much consolidated.

4. Test for preparation. Since the dried tomatoes are normally very pungent, I frequently don't add additional salt. In any case, taste prior to adding additional salt to ensure.

Tips

•Extraordinary with guacamole and salsa, and tortillas for a genuine Mexican dinner.

•In the event that you change the flavoring and leave out the Mexican spice blend however add pcppcr, you can make little meatballs.

•Extraordinary with the pasta marinara.

Tortillas

Fixings
1 cup ground flax seed

1 cup sweet corn (straight from cob or refrozen)
1/2 teaspoon ocean salt
1 cup spring water

Headings

1. Put the corn in a fast blender or food processor and blend well.

2. Add to the bowl with different fixings.

3. Blend all fixings well with a fork, spatula (or hand).

4. Spread meagerly onto teflex sheets or baking paper and put on a baking or parched plate.

5. Dry out at 115° F or 40° C in a dehydrator, hot air stove or in direct daylight for around 4-6 hours.

Tip
•Extraordinary with guacamole or salsa!

Crude French Fries Recipe

Serves 4

Fixings
Fries
4 kohlrabi
1/2 cups cold squeezed olive or hemp seed oil
2 teaspoons curcumin (kurkuma)
1 teaspoon ocean salt

Bearings

1. Cut the kohlrabi resembles french fries (julienne). You can do this with a blade, yet it's most straightforward with a mandolin. There are likewise unique fries cutters you could purchase in the event that you think you'll make this a ton.

2. Put the kohlrabi in a bowl.

3. Put the oil, curcumin and salt in a bowl.

4. Blend and pour over the chips.

5. Let sit for no less than 10 min. Then channel and scoop onto some paper towels (to take off overabundance oil).

Ketchup

3 tomatoes
3 pieces sun dried tomatoes
5 dates (or 1/2 teaspoon stevia and
4 additional sun dried tomatoes)
1 crush lemon juice
1/2 cup unadulterated water

Tip

•Put all fixings in a blender. On the lower part
of the blender the water, lemon juice
furthermore, tomatoes, on top the dried
tomatoes and dates.

•Mix well. This will be simpler on the off
chance that you leave the sun dried tomatoes sit
in water for a
scarcely any hours.

Crude Broccoli Salad

Serves 8

Fixings
1/4 pound broccoli

1 pack scallions (green parts just) finely slashed
(discretionary)
1 cup crude fragmented almonds
1 cup crude sprouted hemp seed
Dressing:
1 cup sesame oil
juice of 1 lemon
1 clove of minced garlic
1 little tranquility of minced ginger
1/4 teaspoon stevia (o 2 tablespoons honey)
1 tablespoon of tamari (discretionary)

Bearings

1. Cut the broccoli into dainty strips as you
would cabbage for coleslaw.

2. Throw the broccoli, scallions, fragmented
almonds and hemp seeds together in an
enormous
bowl and put away.

3. To momentarily make the dressing, put all
the fixings in a blender and mix.

4. Pour the dressing over the serving of mixed
greens and throw to consolidate.

Potato Salad

The best Potato salad. Here is the crude and veggie lover rendition (replaces chicken, potato and mayonnaise).

serves 2-4

Fixings

2 stems celery (cut in minuscule shapes)
1/2 cup pecans (splashed for around 2 hours), cut in quarts
3 apples, cut in little 3D shapes
2 avocados, cut in enormous solid shapes
1 grapefruit, stripped and totally deprived of every single small skin and white piece. kohlrabi or jicama, in little 3D shapes salt and pepper to taste

Bearings

1. Put all fixings with the exception of 1 avocado in a bowl and blend until very much consolidated.

2. Let's represent around 30 minutes.

3. Add the shapes of the subsequent avocado.

4. Serve right away.

5. Decorate with parsley, bits of grapefruit, tomatoes or potentially lettuce.

Tips
•On the off chance that you're not totally crude, you might need to add artichoke hearts (cooked).
•I ordinarily serve all fixings in discrete dishes. Then, at that point, all
relatives can make their own plate of mixed greens and pick what they like. The children love it along these lines.
•You might add a few non crude fixings, for example, the artichoke hearts for "cooked" individuals/visitors.

Lasagna

serves 2-3

Fixings

2 medium zucchinis
2 tablespoons olive oil
squeeze ocean salt
3 ready tomatoes
new basil, cilantro or potentially spinach leafs.

Course

1. Utilizing a mandolin, cheddar slicer or veggie peeler cut long portions of zucchini (as though you would put them on a barbecue).

2. Put all zucchini strips in a bowl and add olive oil and salt and blend.

3. Let stand to marinate for around 30 minutes. This will mellow the zucchini.

4. Meanwhile, set up the ketchup and veggie lover cheddar. Make around 1/2-1 cup of each.

5. Cut the tomatoes in cuts.

6. Presently, take out the zucchini and put on a paper towel to deplete any unreasonable oil or fluid.

7. In a glass or clay square bowl (like one you'd use for making lasagna) line the base with a layer of zucchini. They ought to cover each other somewhat with the goal that you can scoop them out without your lasagna going to pieces.

8. Then, at that point, add a layer of ketchup, a few cuts of tomato and basil, cilantro or spinach leaves.

9. Add a slime layer or a couple of specks of vegetarian cheddar.

10. Again add a layer of zucchini, ketchup, tomato, green leafs, vegetarian cheddar.

11. Rehash once again. Along these lines all out of 3 layers.

Treats, Cake And Pastry

Energy Bars

Serving: Around 6 bars

Fixings
1 1/2 cups dates (or blend)
1 cup nuts (for example crude cashews, almonds, walnuts, or blend) spot of
salt

Headings

1. Pit the dates and spot into a bowl.

2. Transform the dates into a glue. I utilize a blade and cut them into little pieces. On the off chance that you do it in a blender or food processor, the dates adhere to the knives.

3. Place the nuts in a food processor, hand slicer or do it by hand with a sharp blade or knife. Process them yet don't mix to a powder. The bars taste better with small bits of nuts in them.

4. Add the nuts to the dates and blend. This is least demanding with your hands. Blend until completely joined.

5. Take the raw and make 2 long "snakes".

6. Level the top and edges with a wooden spoon.

7. Cut each "square snake" into 3-4 pieces. You might envelop every one by baking paper (or cling wrap). You might put stickers on the wrap or attract on the paper to truly shock yourself, accomplice or children.

8. Store them in the refrigerator until prepared to eat. They travel well, are an incredible evening bite and fulfill kids assuming that you put them in their lunch box.

Tips
•This is only the essential recipe. Your varieties are boundless.
•Blend dates in with figs, apricots, dried apple, raisins, goji berries or attempt a different mix of nuts.

•It's likewise delightful with hemp seed or sesame seeds. Simply ensure the extents are session 1 1/2 products of the soil nuts.
•Add vanilla, cinnamon, chocolate powder or lemon juice for additional delectable taste.
•Assuming that you find making bars and wrapping them an excessive amount of issue. You can likewise simply roll balls.

Frozen yogurt

serves 4

Fixings
1 cup coconut meat
1 cup cashew nuts
1 teaspoon stevia (or 1/2 cup agave syrup or honey)
1 teaspoon vanilla powder or 1 vanilla bean
run ocean salt

Bearings
1. Put all fixings in a blender and mix until totally smooth.
2. Process through your frozen yogurt producer as indicated by directions (is faster on the off chance that you first cool in refrigerator)

Tips

This is the premise of the frozen yogurt recipe. Your varieties are boundless:

1.   Add products of your choice like strawberries, mango, banana, pear, blueberries.

2. Add lemon juice or crude cacao powder and add more stevia to the recipe.

3. In the event that you can't find coconut, you may likewise supplant the coconut and cashews with 2 cups of new almond milk (or other nut milk).

Vanilla Cream

Serves 3-4

Fixings
2 Cups Coconut Meat
1 Cup Cashew Nuts (discretionary)
1/2 cup Coconut water
1 teaspoon 1/2 cup agave syrup
1 teaspoon vanilla powder or 1 vanilla bean

Headings

1. Put all fixings in a blender and mix until totally smooth.

Tips

This cream makes an extraordinary dessert with new natural products or with no guarantees. You may likewise run it in your ice cream producer for a flavorful rich frozen yogurt.

Smoothie, Milks And Squeezes

Carrot Juice

Fixings

1 lbs huge carrots (washed and stripped)
1/2 lemon (stripped) not many green leafs, for example, red lettuce or carrot greens 1 apple

Headings

1. Put all fixings in your juicer. (a rotator juicer is most straightforward for carrots.)

2. Blend and drink right away.

Tips

I strip the carrot for taste (in any case it tastes excessively hearty). I track down this recipe as adequately sweet, yet, in the event that you're a novice juicer or have a sweet tooth, add an apple for additional pleasantness. The medical advantages of carrot juice? It gives Vitamin A, B Nutrients, Vitamin E and numerous minerals (counting calcium).

Incredible for pregnant and nursing moms, visual perception, bones and teeth, liver and nails, skin and hair as well as assisting in bosom and skin disease with forestalling.

Spinach Vegetable Juice

This juice recipe is ideal first of all for veggie squeezing. It's delicate and sweet. Extremely delectable. Not harsh or solid by any means.

Fixings

1 pack spinach
2 apples
1/2 lemon, stripped (discretionary)
Bearings
Put all fixings in your juicer. A twin stuff juicer like the Green Star
Juicer or slow juicer is best for removing greens.

Tomato Vegetable Juice

Are you searching for the best of all tomato juice recipes! This one is!

You can juice the tomatoes in a juicer yet in the event that you have a high velocity blender -, for example, a Vitamix or Blendec Blender - and you like more "body" to your juice, you could jump at the chance to utilize the blender instead.

Fixings

3 cups slashed tomatoes
1 stem celery
1 cucumber
3 drops stevia (discretionary)
1/2 teaspoon himalaya ocean salt pepper
cayenne pepper

Headings
1. Juice the tomatoes, celery, cucumber in your juicer.
2. Add drops of stevia in the event that you like a better taste, salt, pepper and cayenne pepper to taste.
3. In the event that you like you can likewise add a 1/4 onion, new oregano and basil and red ringer pepper.

Dandelion Apple Smoothie

This yummy recipes is one more #1 of mine. It's perfect with spinach as well. Simply supplant the dandelion with spinach.

Fixings

1 pack dandelion greens 1 lemon (stripped)
2 huge apples
1 banana
2 teaspoons flax seeds (discretionary)
Spring or refined water

Bearings

1. Put all fixings in the blender.

2. Add sufficient unadulterated water so all fixings are covered.

3. You can add a banana for richness (discretionary).

4. Mix well and drink.

Hot cocoa

Serves 1

Fixings
1 cup almond milk made with warm water (up
to 115 F or 45 C)
4 tablespoons crude chocolate powder
1 tablespoon honey or coconut nectar
fluid stevia to taste

Headings

1. Mix the crude chocolate powder and
honey/coconut nectar into a glue.

2. Add the almond milk and mix well. Serve
right away.

Tip
•For more sultry chocolate, make almond milk
with around 50% of how much water. Mix all
the fixings, then, at that point, add 2 cups of
heated water. Whisk and serve.

Alkalize For Wellbeing

How basic your blood is, is a simple method for estimating the level of your wellbeing. A solid individual has a blood pH of 7.365. By and large, an individual who is terminal sick has a pH of around 5 or lower.

What Are Antacid, Corrosive And PH?

Soluble food sources are food sources that raise the amount of oxygen that your blood takes in. The most alkalizing food sources are Crude green verdant vegetables, non-sweet products of the soil wheat grasses. Something contrary to soluble food sources are corrosive food sources.

How much oxygen your blood can retain is estimated on a pH scale that reaches from 0 to 14. A pH of 0 is generally acidic while a pH of 14 is generally basic.

Soluble Food Sources Rundown

During the greater part of your lives, most of the food sources you eat are (exceptionally) acidic. These make you weary. By eating crude basic food varieties and beverages, you can assist your body with mending itself from numerous persistent infections.

When in doubt the accompanying food sources bunches are alkalizing:
•Green verdant vegetables (for example spinach, kale);

•Wild greens (e.g., dandelion, weeds, wild grasses);

•New spices (for example parsley, cilantro, basil, garlic);

•Grasses (for example wheat, grain grass);

•Sprouts;

•Ocean vegetables (for example kelp, nori, dulse, spirulina, blue green growth);

•Therapeutic mushrooms (for example shiitake, maitake, reishi).Corrosive Food varieties Rundown Unfortunately the food varieties you might like most make you generally acidic and accordingly wiped out:

•Garbage and Handled food varieties;

•Sugar;

•All creature food (meat, eggs, chicken, fish, lobster, shellfish);

•Grains: (white) wheat, rice, pasta, flour, bread and so forth.;

•A few Organic products;

•Dairy items (milk, cheddar, margarine);

•Awful fats;

•Peanuts, cashews.

The best antacid beverages are basic water, youthful coconut water, vegetable juice also, and wheatgrass juice. Assuming that you're exceptionally acidic you could require soluble enhancements to get you back in balance speedier.

How Sound Would you say you are?

How would you know your body pH? You just get some pH test strips (likewise called litmus paper) at a wellbeing store and pee on one. The paper will tell you in a split second what your pH is and in this way, how basic or corrosive you are (and how sound).

What Is The PH Scale

PH represents Potential for liberating Hydrogen particles. The contrast between corrosiveness also, alkalinity depends on the capacity to free hydrogen particles. Basically, the pH scale estimates how much oxygen is in your blood.

When your blood is too corrosive it won't convey sufficient oxygen. At the point when it is excessively soluble, it will convey excessively. The scale goes from 0 to 14. A pH of 7 is nonpartisan, a pH of 0-7 is corrosive. A pH of 7-14 is soluble. Every unit of progress addresses a ten times change in sharpness or alkalinity.

Consequently the distinction between a pH of 4 and 5 is a lot more prominent than the distinction between 6 a 7. Hence your blood is in balance when you are marginally basic: a pH of 7.365.

Step By Step Instructions To Kill Unsafe Acids

At the point when you're simply beginning a crude food diet, it could be difficult to become soluble. Regardless of whether you eat crude greens day in and day out. I track down that squeezing (with natural products or spices for taste) speeds up this process immensely, yet it might in any case not be sufficient. In that case, you might need to utilize some alkalizing supplements. Models are (Himalayan) ocean salt, pearl calcium, silica, pH drops, green powder, E3 Live or other super food varieties.

Rundown

The rundown of antacid food is all that is crude and green (particularly greens, ocean vegetables, superfoods and spices) and a corrosive food list is all creature items, grains, sugars, fats and seeds. To remain basic 80% of your food ought to be antacid and 20 acidic.

To test your pH you can purchase pH test strips for not exactly $ 15,- (on the web, wellbeing store or drug store). The test will require 2 seconds.